Live Better Meditation

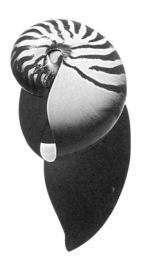

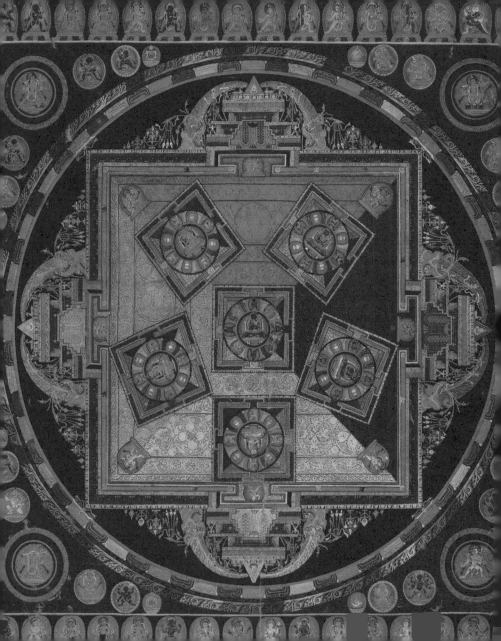

Live Better Meditation

exercises and inspirations for well-being

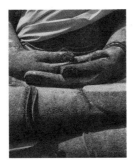

Bill Anderton

DUNCAN BAIRD PUBLISHERS

LONDON

Live Better: Meditation
Bill Anderton

First published in the United Kingdom
and Ireland in 2002 by
Duncan Baird Publishers Ltd
Sixth Floor, Castle House
75–76 Wells Street
London W1T 3QH

Conceived, created and designed by
Duncan Baird Publishers Ltd

Managing Editor: Judy Barratt
Editors: Diana Loxley, with Louise Nixon
Managing Designer: Manisha Patel
Designer: Clare Thorpe
Picture Research: Cee Weston-Baker

British Library Cataloguing-in-Publication Data:
A CIP record for this book is available from the
British Library.

10 9 8 7 6 5 4

ISBN: 1-904292-47-X

Typeset in Filosofia and Son Kern
Colour reproduction by Scanhouse, Malaysia
Printed and bound in Thailand by Sirivatana
Interprint (SI)

Publisher's notes

Before following any advice or practice suggested
in this book, it is recommended that you consult
your doctor as to its suitability, especially if
you suffer from any health problems or special
conditions. The publishers and the author cannot
accept any responsibility for any injuries or
damage incurred as a result of following the
exercises in this book, or of using any of the
therapeutic methods described or mentioned here.

The abbreviations BCE and CE are used throughout
this book. BCE means Before the Common Era
(equivalent to BC); CE means of the Common Era
(equivalent to AD).

contents

INTRODUCTION

If you have always wondered what it would be like to learn to meditate, but have never had the opportunity to try, this book is for you. And, if you have any doubts about whether it is possible to learn to meditate by yourself, and even whether meditation will be effective, let me lay them to rest at the outset.

Meditation is a personal journey, and while it can be helpful to have the reassuring guidance of a teacher, there is nothing about it which prevents you from teaching yourself, with a book such as this as your guide. Some of the benefits of your meditation practice will become clear almost immediately – you may feel calmer, more centred and more focused. Others (such as a deep sense of connection to your inner self, an instinctive harmony with the world around you, and a greater appreciation of your senses) will become clear only over time.

Meditation is an adventure, and like all adventures there may be pitfalls or occasions when progress seems frustratingly slow. Try not to lose heart. Remember:

while it feels right to meditate, it is worth persevering through times of difficulty. However, if at any time on your adventure you feel unhappy about your meditation practice or you feel that it is not in any way beneficial, you should stop. Meditation should never be a cause for discomfort, nor should it be boring or ineffective.

Before embarking upon any journey, it is important to equip yourself properly. This book presents all the essential information you need to set you on your way. First, it hopes to dispel some of the many myths about meditation. Myths such as "meditation makes you lose control of your mind" (it does not – meditation helps to harness control of the mind) and "meditation is really any excuse to do nothing" (on the contrary, outer still-ness can belie the mental energy busily at work at the core of our being). Then, by drawing upon and adapting the meditative traditions of the ancient East, we learn how to practise meditation in a way that is fully in tune with modern times. Meditation is an exciting explo-ration of your own self. Good luck on your journey – may it bring you wisdom and insight for many years to come.

Chapter One

mind and body

To be healthy human beings and to function at the peak of our potential, we need to achieve a balance of mind and body. If we serve our outer needs without allowing ourselves time for the person within, and especially if we ignore the inner voice that tells us to slow down or take a break, then at some point our health will begin to suffer. At the very least, our ability to withstand stress or pressure will be weakened. Meditation is an effective way to ensure that we are not neglecting an important aspect of our well-being – the state of our mind, and its optimum relation with our body.

To achieve this goal, there is no need to spend hours in strict contemplation. A few minutes each day can be enough. Gradually, we will begin to understand the mind–body relationship and in the process discover a new dimension in our lives. By learning to meditate we can even, in due course, tap into a source of healing and rejuvenation deep within ourselves. It is not the amount of time we spend in meditation that counts, but the development of our understanding during that time.

In this chapter we take the first steps toward learning about some of the traditions of meditation, as well as what meditation is and how it is helpful to us; we also examine the basic techniques, such as correct breathing and posture, that will enable us to set off confidently together on our meditation journey.

9

MIND-BODY CONNECTIONS

Far from being isolated, disparate entities, our minds and bodies work together in a relationship of mutual dependency, each drawing support from the other. Only when both are fully nourished can we live balanced and harmonious lives. The way we think and feel about ourselves has a direct influence on our bodies, and *vice versa*: a healthy body will help to create a healthy mind. For example, when athletes reach peak physical fitness, their performance can be further enhanced if the right mental conditions are present to enable them to do so. From a less positive perspective, if you believe in your mind that you are unable to achieve something, then this can have a strong negative influence on your physical ability to do so. Such negative self-images can prevent us from attaining our true potential in life.

Learning to recognize this binding relationship between mind and body can help to change the quality of our lives. Through a process of inner exploration and interpretation, meditation can help you to understand the interconnectedness of the mind and body, and your unconscious thoughts and motivations. The images that come to us in meditation are like dreams: they are born out of the unconscious and correspond with unconscious energies (see pages 44–5). They can be understood in the same way as dream images – they have *symbolic* significance and should not be taken literally. In meditation, unlike dreams, you can delve into and explore these images, letting them change and grow in your mind's eye (see exercise, page 49). Meditation then becomes a creative process in which you allow the symbols that arise from your unconscious into your conscious mind to evolve and reveal their true meaning.

When you meditate everything becomes imbued with significance: "coincidences" seem to have purpose and to have occurred for particular personal reasons. For example, "chance" meetings may be more intimately connected with your unconscious than you had previously thought possible. So, when you meditate, take careful note not only of what happens inside yourself, but also of what happens *to* you.

WHAT IS MEDITATION?

Expressed simply, meditation is the creation of a relaxed state of awareness of mind and body. Under normal circumstances, we experience relaxation and awareness as separate states, not simultaneously, and our concentration is most often directed toward the outside world – for example, when driving a car, our thoughts are focused on what is happening on the road. In meditation, our awareness is directed inward toward our private thoughts and feelings.

Traditional Eastern meditation (see pages 16–17) emphasizes the need to empty the mind of its swirling chatter so as to connect with a greater reality beyond. However, we will be taking a slightly different approach – we will begin not by clearing the mind, but by filling it with a wealth of thoughts, images and feelings. In doing so, we connect more fully with our inner being and develop a deeper understanding of our true nature. We will be meditating not on a higher spiritual realm but, quite simply, on ourselves.

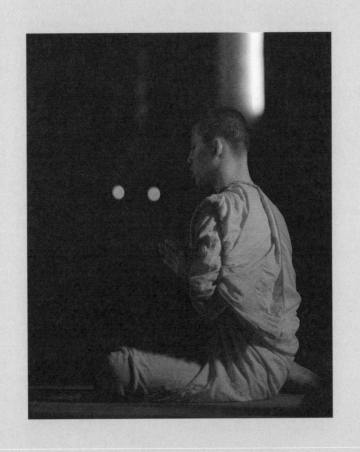

WHY MEDITATE?

People turn to meditation for a variety of reasons. Many are drawn to it because they want to learn to relax and eliminate unnecessary stress and tension in their lives. The effect of meditation can be like taking a holiday — when you return, you are refreshed and re-acquainted with yourself and you have a new perspective on your life and problems. But unlike expensive holidays, meditation costs nothing and needs only a few minutes of your time every day.

Think of the stream of thoughts that endlessly flows through your head all the time you are awake. When you are alone, and your mind is not focused on any particular activity or task, these thoughts will tend to dart in all directions, more or less randomly. The truth is, many of these thoughts will be unconstructive or anxious; they will be tinged with various emotional responses, as if someone had emptied bottles of dye into the stream of your consciousness; they will probably keep you tense or even make you stressed.

Meditation puts us closer in touch with our minds as well as our bodies and helps us to understand our unconscious motives and desires – it enables us to identify negative thoughts and emotions and to work through and eliminate those feelings which are unhelpful to us. Once we discover the unconscious forces operating in our inner lives, we can make changes for the better.

The practical and physical benefits of meditation are well recognized. Correct breathing, good posture and deep relaxation encourage the body to function more efficiently and can help relieve problems such as insomnia, high blood pressure and low energy levels. Meditate in a spirit of open-mindedness and you will find that you have a clearer understanding of how your body works and who you are. You will probably start to feel more relaxed, and be able to concentrate better. You may even see your problems in a clearer perspective. In connecting with the reality at the deeper levels of your mind, you will burn off the haze of illusion. You will see what it is to be human, and therefore come to appreciate other people more. You will see the connectedness of all life.

TRADITIONS OF MEDITATION

Although we tend to think of meditation as being epito-mized by the holy men of Buddhism, it is in fact central to many of the world's major spiritual and philosophical traditions. Here is a taste of how meditation fits into practices other than Buddhism.

Hinduism

India has long been associated with the quest for spiri-tual enlightenment. Yoga, a practical path to spiritual progress, has been a major focus of the country's reli-gious life for many centuries. It recommends discipline of the body and concentration of the mind (through meditation) as a means to achieving self-realization and enlightenment. Yoga is revered in the sacred texts of Hinduism: for example, the *Bhagavad Gita* (6th century BCE) describes yoga as offering a solution to the prob-lems of life; similarly, yoga is central to the *Upanishads* (*c*.800–*c*.300BCE), which view mind, body, spirit and world as a continuum, a whirling force of life energy.

Taoism

The *Tao Te Ching* – the principle text of Taoism, written by Lao Tsu around the 4th century BCE – is full of wisdom and poetry that speaks to our inner being and teaches that we should accept the world as it is. Taoist philosophy centres on the relationship between opposites: the inner and outer worlds, the conscious and unconscious self. The union of opposites is epitomized in the symbol *yin-yang*. Meditation is recommended as the means of achieving order and unity in our own life.

Celtic Christianity

Celtic Christianity placed great emphasis on the human need for solitude and isolation. Its practitioners would seek out special places in the natural world – perhaps a mountain, or a site near trees or running water, or by the sea – where, through meditation, they could celebrate God and nature as one. Celtic Christians composed many prayers for special occasions that could be repeated over and over again – in a similar fashion to the Buddhist *mantra* (see pages 90–91).

Empty yourself of everything:
Let your mind be at peace.
While ten thousand things rise and fall
the Self contemplates their return.
Each of them grows and flourishes and
then returns to the source.
To return to the source is stillness,
which is to fulfil the way of nature.
The way of nature is constant.
Knowing constancy is insight.

LAO TSU

TAO TE CHING (4TH CENTURY BCE)

THE RIGHT TIME

It is helpful to establish a routine in
meditation – try to put aside a particular time
each day so that meditation practice becomes a
part of your life. Experiment to find out what
suits you best: some people find it refreshing
to meditate at the beginning of the day;
others prefer to practise in the evening,
to calm the mind before bedtime.

THE RIGHT PLACE

Find a quiet place to meditate where you won't
be interrupted. Make this place special by putting
meditation objects, such as cushions, candles and
incense there. Music has a wonderful calming
influence – bear this in mind when choosing your
space. Meditating outside in the open air, so that you
are able to use nature as a focus for your thoughts, can
bring you a deep sense of connection
with the world at large.

HOW TO SIT

Traditional forms of meditation are practised in particular postures, but these can sometimes be uncomfortable and difficult to achieve for the Western body. You don't have to be young and supple to meditate properly – everyone can benefit. For the meditations in this book, the most important thing is to feel comfortable.

Assume a comfortable sitting or lying position. If lying down, you may need a support for your head; if sitting on a chair, make sure that your chair will support your back so that your spine is straight. When sitting on the floor, try to sit cross-legged resting your buttocks on the front edge of a special meditation cushion (or firm pillow). It is important that you are able to breathe freely – sitting with a straight back helps to prevent any restriction of your diaphragm and lungs.

During meditation, the body's metabolism slows down and you may begin to feel cold, so make sure that the room is warm before you begin. Wear loose clothing and remove any obtrusive jewelry.

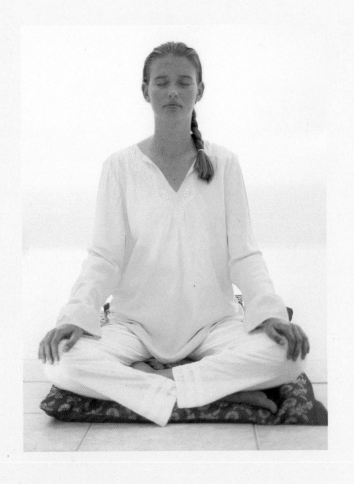

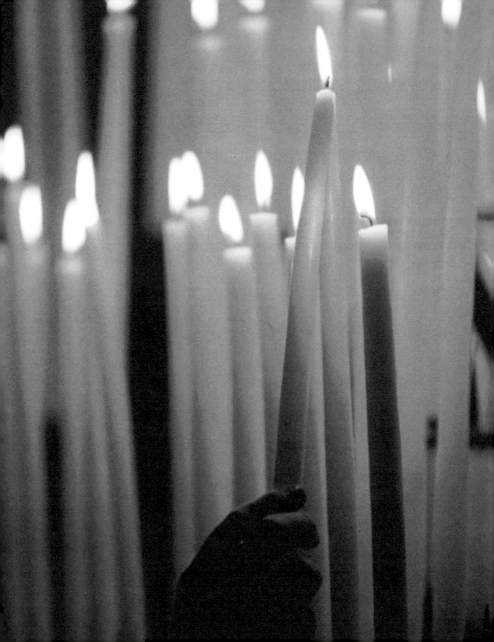

CANDLE MEDITATION

This simple technique helps to settle the mind and provides a good focus for meditation.

1 Sit in a comfortable meditation posture with a lighted candle in front of you. Breathe evenly and a little more deeply than normal. Concentrate your attention on each part of your body in turn, saying to yourself, "I relax easily and completely." Focus your awareness on the flame: imagine that it enters your being and feel that it becomes a part of you.

2 Close your eyes, but hold the image of the candle and flame in your mind's eye. Carry the image into the depths of your mind. As you absorb inwardly the mental picture of the candle flame, lose any sense of its separateness – you interfuse with the flame as the flame interfuses with your being.

3 When you are ready, end the meditation by focusing on your breathing once more – breathe a little more deeply for one or two minutes, and then open your eyes.

BREATH AND MEDITATION

Most of us are not conscious of how our breathing affects our physical and mental states, but in meditation observing the breath and the way in which we breathe are crucial. On a purely practical level, if we absorb oxygen and expel waste gases freely, our metabolic system functions efficiently – this, in turn, enables our body to relax. Just taking a few moments to fill our lungs and steady our breathing can calm us greatly in times of stress and tension. Meditation teaches us that, by learning to understand and regulate our breathing, we can develop the ability to control our bodies, focus our minds and control our emotions and thereby improve the overall quality of our lives.

Correct breathing is fundamentally linked with correct posture – this not only makes us look good but, far more importantly, helps us to feel good too. When sitting, make sure that your back is straight, but not tense. If you meditate in a cramped position, your lungs and diaphragm will not be able to move or expand freely and easily. Effective breathing comes from deep in the diaphragm, not from the upper chest.

Try to establish a routine in your meditation sessions: when you first close your eyes and prepare to meditate, make it a habit that the next thing you do is focus your attention on your breathing. For a minute or two, try to breathe slowly, evenly and a little more deeply than you would normally. This will automatically help you to relax and to still your mind. Contemplate the process of breathing and how your very existence depends upon it, and you will alert yourself to the importance it plays in your health and well-being. When we breathe we are taking in the surrounding air and making it a part of ourselves. Contemplation of this process makes us aware of the close and binding relationship we have with our environment. In fact, focusing on our breathing is a meditation in itself.

End each meditation in the same way that you begin it: just before opening your eyes and finishing your meditation, spend a minute or two concentrating on every inhalation and every exhalation as they occur.

RELAXING YOUR BODY

Use this meditation sequence, along with the breathing technique described on pages 26–7, to help you to enter a state of relaxed awareness.

1 Sit or lie comfortably on the ground with your legs stretched out in front of you. Begin your meditation, as always, by breathing freely, easily and deeply.

2 Concentrate on relaxing each part of your body in turn, beginning with your feet, then your legs, lower body, chest, arms, back, shoulders, and ending with your facial muscles. As you meditate, repeat to yourself, "I am feeling more and more relaxed."

3 If you are a light, airy person, imagine that your whole body feels heavy; if you are a heavy, earthy person, imagine that your body feels light. Concentrate on the feeling for as long as you feel comfortable.

4 Finally, refocus on your breathing. When you are ready, open your eyes to end the meditation.

RELEASING DISCOMFORT

Discomfort can sometimes arise during meditation. If this is because of muscle tension, try tightening up the muscle concerned, and then releasing it – imagine that the tension flows out of you like a stream. Alternatively, focus your awareness on the area of discomfort, but do nothing else – simply allow the sensation to pass through your mind and drift away (this approach is not recommended for the elderly or the infirm). If you experience a tingling sensation in your body, adopt a more comfortable position to allow your blood to circulate more freely.

OPENING YOUR EYES

Open your eyes at any time during meditation if you feel uneasy with them closed. Try to stay completely relaxed when you do this so that you retain your state of meditative awareness. When you are ready, simply close your eyes again.

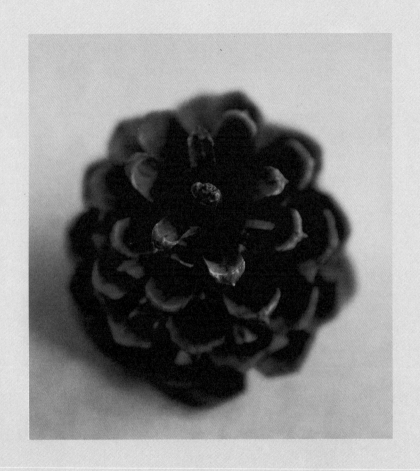

DEVELOPING FOCUS

The underlying key to meditation is learning how to "centre" ourselves – how to still our bodies and focus our minds so that we are able to enter a state of total absorption and concentration. Try putting your personal preoccupations on hold and direct your awareness to whatever item you may want to let your attention rest on. You may wish to focus on a specific part of your body by chanelling all your mental energy there. Or you may want to place a particular object or image – perhaps a flower, vase or painting – in front of you and allow your eyes gently ro rest on it as a point of focus. Initially, you may find that your concentration lies solely on the chosen object; in time, your thoughts and your object of thought will become as one.

The ability to concentrate for long periods during meditation is an enriching experience, but don't worry if at first you are distracted and your thoughts dart in all directions – try to bring them back into focus and, with practice, your powers of concentration will increase.

As well as developing your focus and awareness, you must centre yourself to achieve a sense of mental and physical balance. In Zen Buddhism, the area from the abdomen down to the groin is known as the *hara*. Within this area, about five centimetres (two inches) below the navel, is the *tanden* – a point said to be the exact centre of gravity and the point of balance for the entire body. Focusing your thoughts on the *tanden* during meditation should help you to develop a greater sense of physical and mental equilibrium.

Meditation should not be regarded as something you do for a few minutes each day – it is an attitude that can be carried through into your everyday life. Practise centring your mind and body, and you will find it will have a profound effect on the way you live your daily life, enabling you to stay focused on whatever task you set yourself, and allowing you to absorb yourself totally in every aspect of your physical, mental and emotional existence. When we clear our minds and still our bodies – even if only for a short while – we attract rich and subtle blessings into our lives.

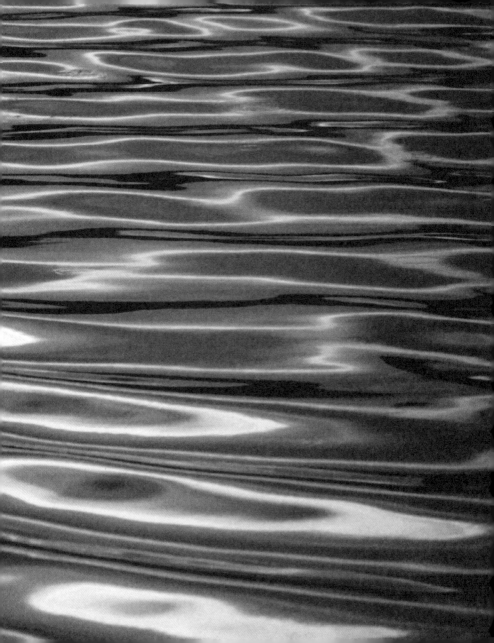

STILLING YOUR MIND

This exercise will help you to still your mind by monitoring your thoughts as they come and go.

1 Sit in your meditation position. Relax, breathe naturally and easily, and focus your attention on your thoughts. Don't stop or censor your thoughts — allow them to flow freely in and out of your consciousness. Imagine that your thoughts are ripples on a pond. Be patient and you should eventually feel enveloped in stillness.

2 When you feel calm, centre your mind on the word "peace". Meditate on this word. Let it fill your mind and body, and allow it to resonate through you.

3 After two to three minutes, release the word so that only the essence of peace (the physical sense of its presence) remains within you.

4 At the end of your meditation, notice how relaxed you feel — try to hold on to this feeling. Breathe a little more deeply for a minute and then open your eyes.

There is one thing that, when cultivated
and regularly practised, leads to
deep spiritual intention, to peace, to
mindfulness and clear comprehension,
to vision and knowledge, to a happy
life here and now, and to the
culmination of wisdom and awakening.
And what is that one thing?
It is mindfulness centred on the body.

THE BUDDHA

(c.563–c.483BCE)

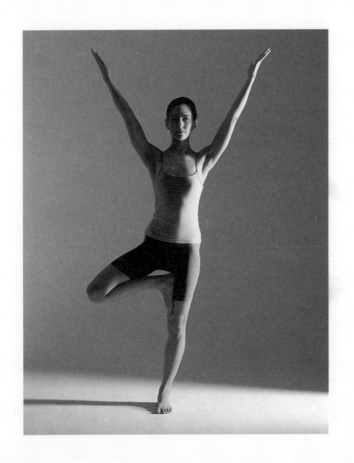

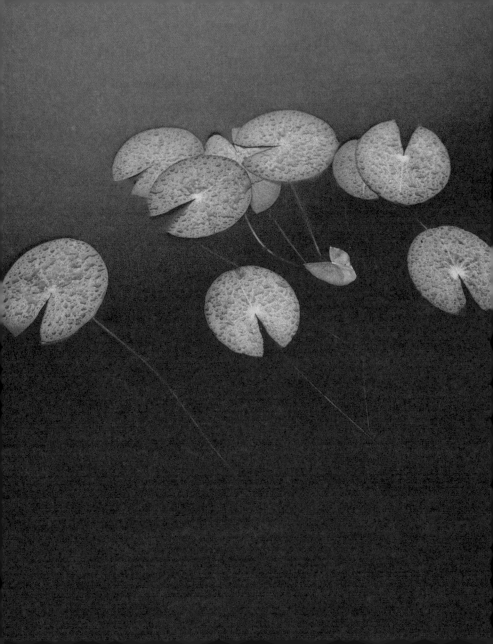

CENTRE YOURSELF

This exercise shows you how to develop a still, quiet mind and a firm, steady body – both of which are important prerequisites for effective meditation.

1 Sit in a comfortable position with your back straight. Roll your shoulders back to broaden your chest. Place your hands, palms down, on your knees or thighs. Close your eyes. Focus on your body, releasing any muscles that feel tense. Keep your breathing soft and steady.

2 Allow your mind to settle on the innate stability and strength of your inner self. If other thoughts start drifting into your mind, gently try to return the focus to your breathing – inhaling for strength, exhaling for stability.

3 Return your awareness to the physical presence of your body: notice the air against your skin, the weight of your body as it touches the floor or your chair, the warmth of your toes, the light touch of your hair against your face. Sit quietly for a few moments, consolidating this awareness of yourself, before getting up.

MEDITATING "PROPERLY"

People are often unsure whether or not they are
meditating "properly". The answer to this is that,
strictly speaking, there is no right or wrong way – it
depends entirely on what you want to achieve through
your practice. If meditation does not appear to be
helping you in any way, there may be something you
need to change. Sometimes you can find out what you
need to change on an inner, spiritual level, by
listening to the voice of your unconscious. While
meditating, try asking yourself what you are aiming
to gain from the practice. Observe the thoughts
and feelings that arise in response.

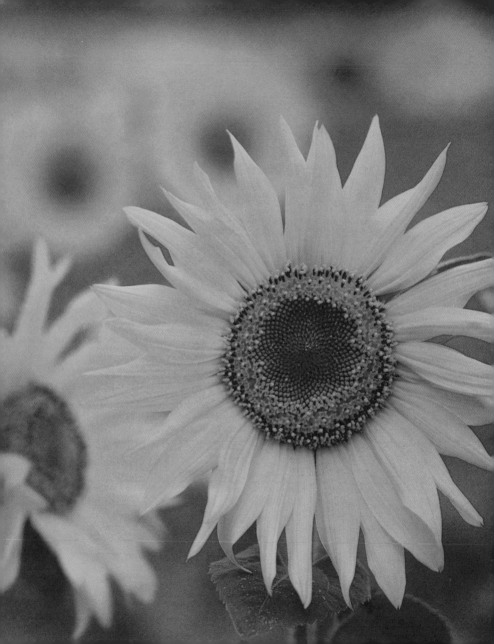

Chapter Two

first steps

Having familiarized ourselves with the basic principles and techniques of meditation, we are now equipped to delve more deeply into the mental and spiritual resources that we will need to draw upon as we set off on our journey. At this stage, we should recognize that meditation can become a way of life – sitting down and focusing your mind is just a small part of the experience. You may discover that change arises naturally in all areas of your life when you introduce meditation. And although you do not necessarily need to alter your lifestyle dramatically to benefit from meditation, a certain level of commitment is desirable. The extent of this commitment is entirely up to you.

In this chapter we explore, among other things, the concept of "mindfulness" – that is, of giving our full attention and awareness to the thoughts and feelings that take place in our minds and bodies. For example, we can become "mindful" of the instinctive drives that control our eating habits, our attitude to exercise, or our abuse of our bodies through smoking and drinking. By fully encountering these drives and impulses and becoming more conscious of them, we take a step toward improving the quality of our lives.

Begin your meditation journey with an open mind. Have no expectations. Be patient and welcome any positive changes that come into your life.

MEETING YOUR MIND

The mind constantly plays tricks on us and has many strategies for distracting our attention, setting us on the wrong path, deceiving us and leading us astray. This trickster may appear in the form of negative thoughts that try to prevent us from achieving a goal – the harder we try to succeed, the more obstructive our thoughts might become. Take note of the tactics your mind adopts to pull you away from your chosen path. Your mind may intervene during meditation to tell you that you are wasting your time or that the practice is not working – it could do anything to divert you from your mental goal.

Obstructive thoughts stem from the unconscious mind – that part of ourselves which determines much of what motivates us: our desires, impulses and instincts. If we fail to engage with our unconscious, then we are ignoring a fundamental part of our innermost being. The unconscious contains both negative and positive aspects: but while these remain unconscious, they can be neither encouraged nor discouraged.

The conscious mind is like a light which can be shone into the unconscious to reveal the mind's hidden contents. Meditation teaches us how gradually to become better acquainted with the mechanisms of our unconscious mind and how to make our unconscious thoughts conscious, for our own eventual benefit. It is through this marriage of opposites – a communion of the conscious and unconscious minds – that we are able to enhance our self-knowledge and self-awareness.

One of the first things to take into account when encountering your mind is that people are all different. Although we all have similar needs (such as the need for food, warmth and shelter) and experience similar emotions (for example, love, hate, fear and desire), our individual histories and psychological make-up diverge widely and define our characters in different ways. In meditation, this means that what may be effective for one person may not work for another. Bear this in mind when choosing and practising your meditation exercises – experiment to find out what works best for you and what you feel most comfortable with.

MINDFULNESS

Western culture tends to place great value on individual wealth and the outward signs of "success" without recognizing the value of a rich inner, spiritual life. It has created a frenzied, goal-driven environment in which it is increasingly difficult to find the opportunity to focus on individual thoughts, feelings and actions or to contemplate our relationship with the world around us. Eastern tradition offers a radical alternative to the materialism of the modern age and has much to teach us about the nature of "being". When subtly adapted to suit our modern lives, Eastern philosophy can help us to rediscover the spiritual values sadly lacking in our modern Western lifestyles.

The full awareness of our movements and sensations, our actions, emotions and thoughts is referred to in Zen Buddhism as "mindfulness". It is the process of placing the mind firmly in the present and keeping it totally absorbed in the task that is being performed. Meditation, in which the mind becomes fully alert, is itself a mindful activity. As adults, one of the skills we tend to lose is that of giving our experiences our full attention. As we walk along, wrapped up in our thoughts, our senses seem often to be only half awake to our surroundings – to the sights, sounds and smells that bombard us from all directions. We also tend to forget the ways our breath and our body feel to us, and we may not even be fully aware of our thoughts or our emotions. To be wholly engaged in every aspect of our physical, mental and emotional existence is to be mindful.

The concept of mindfulness takes on even greater relevance when we learn – perhaps contrary to the traditional approach to meditation – not to vanquish the contents of our minds, but to observe them, to shine the light of awareness on them and illuminate their significance. A major stumbling block for many people who try to follow the teachings of traditional meditation is that they find it impossible to empty their minds. But to empty the mind is to deny its reality – only when we encounter it fully and take heed of its contents, can we begin to experience the richness of life to the full.

DISCOVERING YOUR IMAGINATION

In this exercise a box is used as a focus for your meditation. As you visualize the box, let your imagination take over. Allow items in the box to "appear" – these represent your thoughts and feelings.

1 It may help to place an empty box in front of you and observe it for a few moments. When you are ready, close your eyes and picture the box in your mind's eye.

2 Imagine that the box represents your mind, and you open it to discover that it contains certain objects. What do you see inside the box? Are there items that represent your life, your personality or your mood? Perhaps there are random objects that don't seem to make sense – they could be messages from your unconscious.

3 Imagine removing each item from the box. What feelings does each item arouse in you? Accept your feelings, whatever they might be. To end the meditation, imagine placing the items back in the box, and closing the lid. Take a few deep breaths and open your eyes.

LIVING IN THE PRESENT

Meditation encourages us to focus the mind
and concentrate our mental energies. If we
are constantly dwelling on the past or
worrying about the future, we hinder our
ability to be fully aware of the present.
Meditation encourages us to awaken to the
reality of today and, in so doing, offers us
freedom not only from all that has been but
also from all that will be.

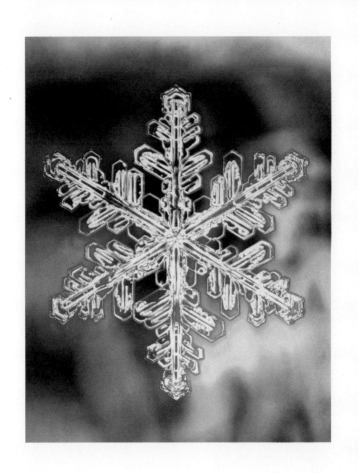

MONITORING YOUR THOUGHTS

Thinking involves making associations, letting our thoughts and imagination expand and develop freely and naturally. In meditation, not only do we have to use our imagination and our ability to think, but we also need to be able to monitor the various thoughts and feelings that arise spontaneously in us.

Try detaching yourself and observing the thoughts, images and ideas that flow in and out of you. Imagine they are clouds drifting across the sky. As you watch these thoughts, let them pass through your mind without engaging with them. Do not influence or judge them. Simply be aware of them. Notice the calming effect as you enjoy these quiet moments of observation and reflection. What better way could there be to spend a few minutes than in the observation of your thoughts in a spirit of positive acceptance?

Sometimes during meditation you may find yourself distracted. If this is the case, go with the distraction for a moment or two then gently discipline yourself to return to the focus of your attention. The key is to be passive, aware, non-judgmental and patient. If you feel disappointed with the result of a meditation, then you are being judgmental. Expect nothing. Assume nothing. Open yourself up to all possibilities.

Consider what thoughts and feelings preoccupy you during the day. Try to identify them and write them down. Do you expend a great deal of energy worrying about what will happen in the future or what has happened in the past? Are you often preoccupied with trying to control events or situations over which you have no control? Perhaps you often experience negative feelings (such as anger, hate, regret, fear, sadness) or negative thoughts, such as "Nobody cares what happens to me" or "No one pays any attention to what I do"? Maybe your thoughts are daydreams and you find yourself wishing you were somewhere else, or with someone else, or in a different occupation? Become an observer of your thoughts and learn to identify your thought patterns – gradually introduce this routine not just into your meditation sessions, but into all areas of your daily life.

MIND IMAGES

Using our imagination in meditation enables us to
focus clearly and to delve more deeply into our
innermost thoughts and feelings. Meditate on a
sound or an image and observe closely the effect that it
has on you. All of us have the ability to conjure up and
hold images in our mind's eye, but if you find it
difficult, perhaps your imagination is out of practice.
Persevere, and you will find that making mental
images becomes easier with time.

BUILDING BRIDGES

Allow images in your mind to grow and change,
and to take on a life of their own. Think of this as your
unconscious painting a magnificent masterpiece for
you every day. When you work with your imagination
during meditation, you are building a bridge to your
unconscious. Crossing this bridge will bring you to a
greater realization of your full creative potential.

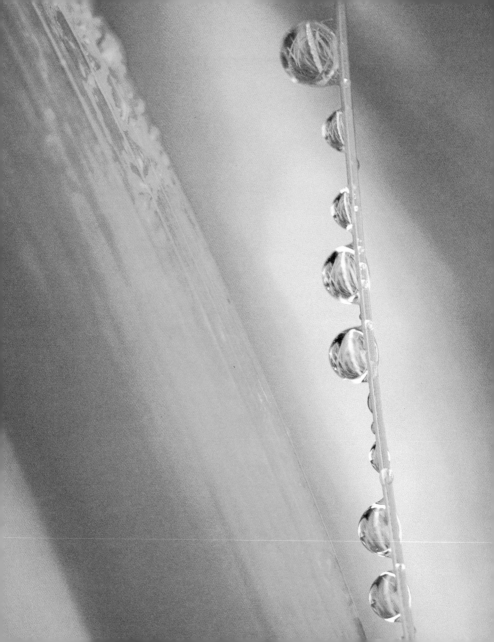

WATCHING YOUR EMOTIONS

It is quite common to experience strong emotions during meditation. If you are by nature an emotional person this may not be a problem for you because you are used to experiencing high levels of feeling, but if you are a cool, unemotional type who is used to keeping their feelings in check, coming face-to-face with your emotions may be a shock. Be prepared for this eventuality.

Rather than being caught up and pushed around by our emotions so that they overwhelm or govern us, through meditation we can learn to observe our emotions and then to understand their nature and to discover why they are occurring. In these ways, we can learn to manage our lives more calmly and rationally – not by turning our feelings on and off at will, but by becoming more aware of them and understanding how best to encounter them and respond to them. Fighting to suppress our emotions or to gain control over them is usually futile. The struggle can often be stressful and tiring, and it is rarely of any psychological benefit.

Our emotions help us to form relationships and in meditation we are learning to develop a relationship with our inner selves. When you experience strong emotions in meditation, monitor how they affect you and whether the feelings are negative or positive. Become an observer of your emotions, not only in meditation but in your daily life. Try to detect patterns in the way you react to situations, and find out what the triggers are.

If you have a well of strong, overwhelming emotion inside you that you want to release, try to let it out gradually and express it in a constructive way – writing about or even drawing a representation of the feeling can be therapeutic and will help you to understand it better. You need to be able to step back from your emotions. If you discover that you are being taken over by them, you should stop and try to let them die down. A good way to deal immediately with powerful emotions, such as rage or burning desire, is to close your eyes and imagine that you are being soothed by a gentle shower of cooling rain. In doing so, you may feel your inner turmoil gradually being washed away.

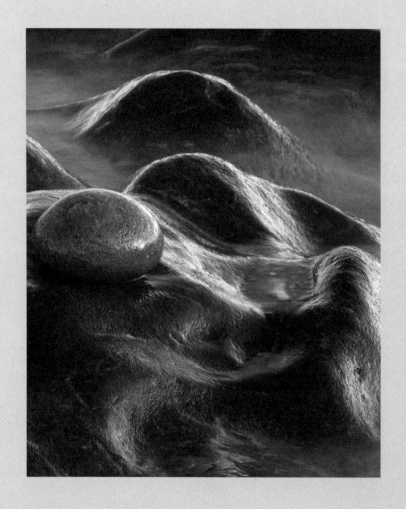

OVERCOMING NEGATIVE EMOTIONS

This exercise will help you to deal with overwhelming or negative emotions that may arise at any time, but especially during meditation.

1   Close your eyes and breathe deeply for a few minutes. When you feel calm, imagine that you are holding a large stone, rock or crystal in your hand. This is your "worry stone". What is its texture and colour?

2   Now bring to mind the negative emotion that you wish to control or dispel. Imagine that you channel this emotion along your arm, down through your hand and fingers, and into the stone, which is able to absorb it.

3   Visualize the stone absorbing all the thoughts that trigger a negative emotional response in you. Allow the stone to soak up these thoughts until you sense that they are dying down and ceasing to trouble you.

4   When the thoughts (and your emotions) have receded, imagine that you wash the stone to cleanse it – in doing so, you wash away all your negative emotional energy.

Breathing in, I see myself as a mountain.
Breathing out, I feel solid.
Breathing in, I see myself as space.
Breathing out, I feel free.

THICH NHAT HANH
(20TH CENTURY)

Things of the past are already gone.
and things to be distant beyond imagining.
The Tao is just this moment, these words:
plum blossoms fallen; gardenia just opening.

CH'ING KUNG
THE MOUNTAIN DWELLING (14TH CENTURY)

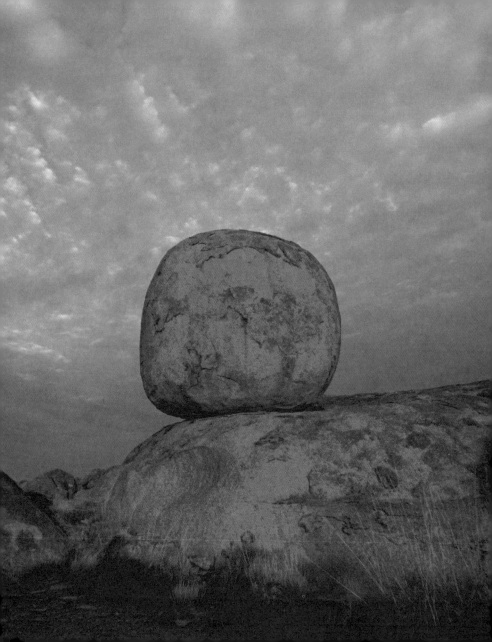

MINDFULNESS OF THE BODY

We tend not to pay full attention to our body unless we are experiencing physical pain or discomfort. It is almost as though we walk around all day attached to our body, making it work for us, but without really being aware of its existence. Mindfulness involves learning to become more aware of our body as well as of our thoughts and feelings (see pages 46–7).

Think for a moment about how conscious you are of your body as you go about your daily business. Become aware of the different sensations you have – the contact of your feet with the floor; your torso's contact with a chair or cushions (or both); the sensations of air against your skin; and, deeper, the movements of your muscles and ligaments. Meditation encourages us to be more mindful of the relationship that exists between our mind and our body and of how our thoughts and emotions affect us physically. Awareness and nurturing of this relationship will have a fundamental impact on our spiritual and physical well-being.

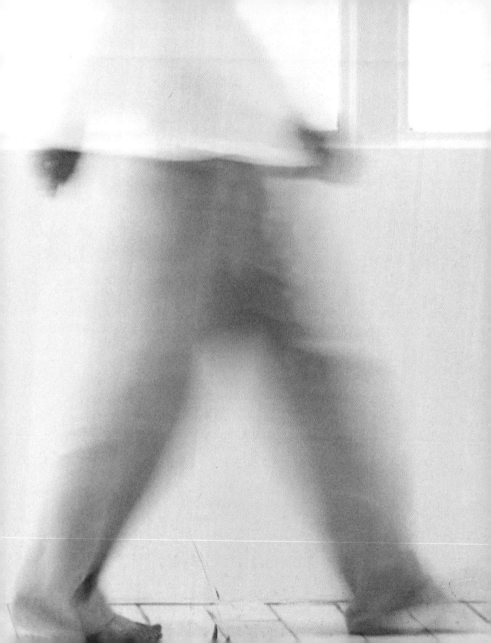

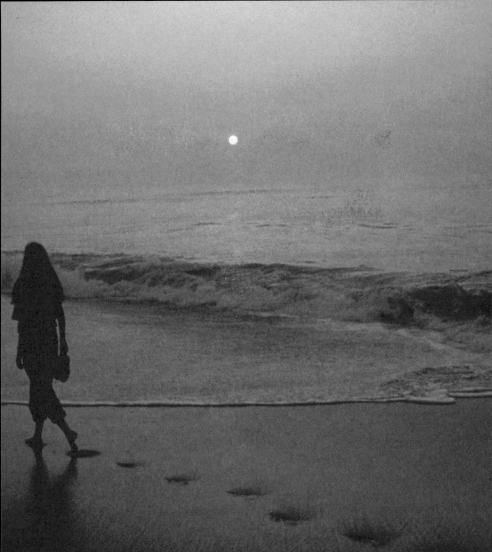

WALKING MEDITATION

Practised regularly the following exercise (based on *kinhin*, a Zen meditation technique) will increase your awareness of the relationship between your mind and body. Practise it for as long as you feel comfortable.

1 Find a peaceful space, preferably outdoors. Choose a place where you can walk freely for a few minutes without having to negotiate your way round too many obstacles and without being disturbed by other people.

2 Walk steadily at a slow and deliberate pace. Focus on each part of your body in turn, beginning at your feet and working upward, and note how each part feels. Observe how you can control the way in which each part of your body contributes to the process of walking.

3 Let this experience be a calming one — allow your thoughts to come and go as you focus on the act of walking. Ensure that you are fully aware of how it feels to be "in" your body. When you feel ready, return your awareness to the outside world to end the meditation.

The totally awakened warrior can
freely utilize all elements contained
in heaven and earth. The true warrior
learns how to perceive correctly the
activity of the universe and how to
transform martial techniques into
vehicles of purity, goodness and
beauty. A warrior's mind and body
must be permeated with enlightened
wisdom and deep calm.

MORIHEI UESHIBA
THE ART OF PEACE (20TH CENTURY)

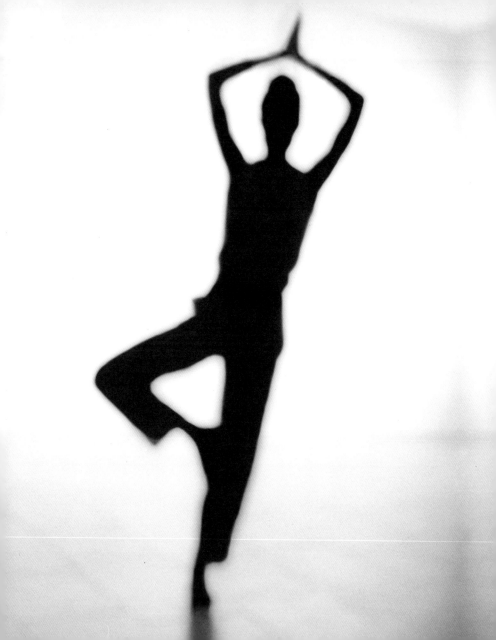

image and sound

All forms of meditation make positive use of our senses of sight and hearing to help us explore our inner being, free our minds and open ourselves up to the possibility of change. In meditation we are creating a relationship between our conscious and unconscious minds, between our everyday world and the realities that lie beyond it. Stimulated and encouraged by different sounds and images, our imagination can be used to form a bridge between these two worlds.

Images and sounds have tremendous creative power contained within them and those used in meditation have been carefully chosen for their ability to expand our consciousness and influence our minds in positive ways.

Certain images and sounds used in meditation are well-known and have evolved over many thousands of years. For example, *mandalas* (geometric representations of the cosmos), help the meditator to achieve a sense of peaceful integration with the universe (see page 73). Similarly, *mantras*, words or phrases chanted in meditation, promote feelings of harmony and well-being.

The following pages show how your senses of sight and hearing can be put to great effect in your meditation sessions. Not only can you make use of traditional images or sounds, but you can also try creating your own – personal tools such as these will hold particular significance for you and will help you to grow spiritually.

THE POWER OF SYMBOLS

The creative force of our imagination is constantly
called upon when we use objects, images and sounds as
focal points for the mind. Encouraging these stimuli to
develop in our mind's eye in meditation is a way to
improve our powers of perception so that we can reach
beyond the bounds of the conscious mind. Objects,
images and sounds can become symbols of something
deeper – reflections of a metaphorical, universal language that lies deep within.

The power of a symbol lies in its ability to epitomize
several ideas at once – even ideas that seem opposite or
contradictory. For this reason we are able to respond to a
symbol on many levels, and our relationship with a particular symbol can grow and change. The all-encom-
passing nature of symbols makes them highly useful as
tools in meditation. Over the following pages we look at
the traditional symbols of *mandalas*, *chakra*s and the
Kabbalah, and draw upon their meanings to help us
make further progress on our meditation journey.

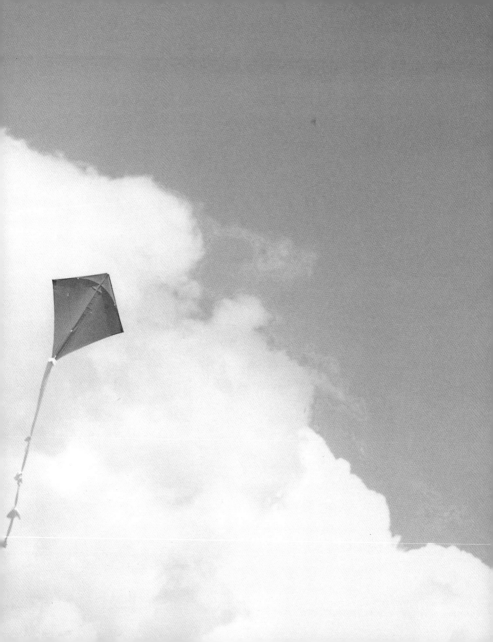

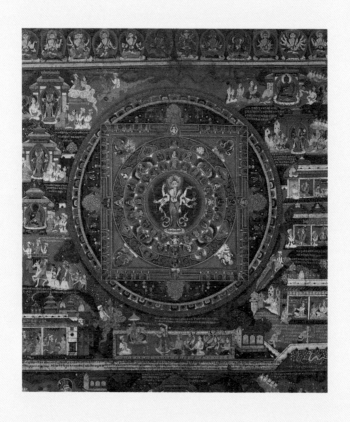

MANDALAS

A *mandala* is a complex, decorative and symmetrical diagram, designed as an aid to meditation and used traditionally in the meditation practices of Hinduism and Buddhism. It is charged with religious symbolism and represents cosmic forces in the form of divine beings. The *mandala* usually has a circular outline which contains a square or squares. The circle represents wholeness and healing; the square is a reminder of divisions and opposites within the whole; the centre, the *mandala*'s focal point, symbolizes the unity of all things.

When you use a *mandala*, you need not be specific in your interpretation of its meaning. As you meditate on it, the *mandala* can bring a profound sense of harmony – a mystical sense of oneness with the cosmos. The best approach is to focus on it without concerning yourself with its deep spiritual significance. You can do this by entering into the images, like someone entering a room and taking in its features – but not judging them – in a state of mental alertness, or mindfulness.

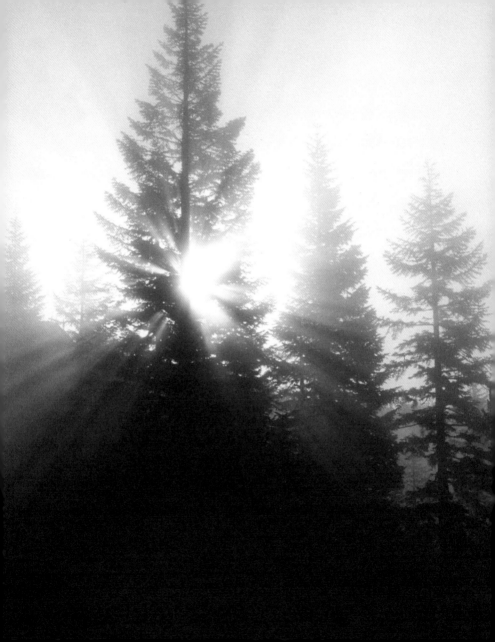

HEALING VISUALIZATION

In this exercise we draw upon the cosmic, symbolic principles of the *mandala* to create our own unifying visualization. This meditation is a good one to practise if you are feeling "disconnected" from the world, or generally under par.

1 Sit comfortably, close your eyes and relax. In your mind's eye, picture a cross within a circle – this is a universal symbol of healing and wholeness. Imagine that each of the four quarters of the circle is like a window. Look through each window in turn. Try to paint or create a picture in each window. Create whatever comes to you.

2 Imagine that the cross in the circle begins to radiate a healing light that grows in intensity. As you continue to meditate on the light, it radiates out from the circle and fills your whole mind and body with its brilliance.

3 When you are ready to end the meditation, let the light die down and the image of the circle fade. Breathe a little deeper, stay completely relaxed and open your eyes.

THE CHAKRAS

Western medicine tends to view the body as a collection of disparate parts, many of which can be treated in isolation from one another. Other traditions view the body in a more holistic way, recognizing an essential inner energy, or life force. According to yogic tradition, the body has a system of *chakras*, or energy centres, which cannot be seen physically, but are positioned along the line of the spine. Many Indian healers describe them as "spinning wheels of energy".

In the traditional Hindu texts, the *chakras* are associated with particular animals, birds, gods and goddesses, whose attributes help to describe the qualities and properties (such as humility, strength and loving compassion) of the different *chakras*. Each *chakra* is represented by a *mandala*-like diagram, and is also associated with a colour and a part or parts of the body. When meditating on *chakras*, we are encouraged to focus on their associations, explore their qualities and direct "energy-flow" toward them.

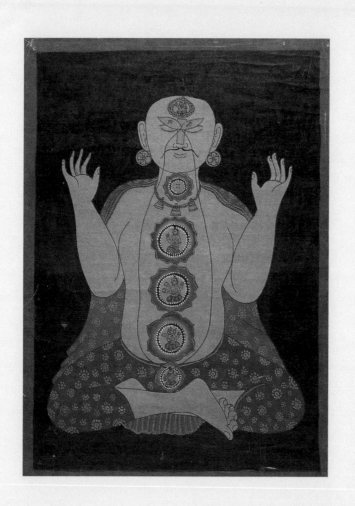

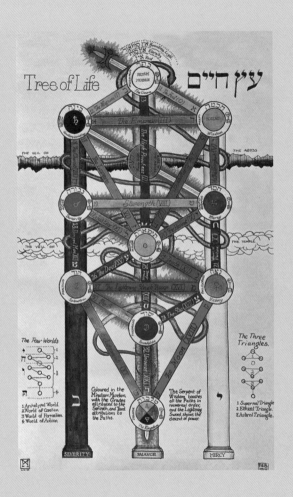

Tree of Life עץ חיים

THE KABBALAH

Originally a body of teachings associated with the Jewish mystical tradition, the Kabbalah has evolved over the 2,000 years or so of its history into a living tradition relevant to the 21st century. Adapted by the Western esoteric practices of modern magic – most noticeably, the Hermetic Order of the Golden Dawn – the Kabbalah gained a reputation for being dark and mysterious. But today its teachings are open and available to all. Of particular interest is its guidance on the discovery of spiritual knowledge through meditation.

The Kabbalah uses a model or map called the Tree of Life to describe its teachings. A symbol of cosmic unity, the tree, or *sephiroth*, is made up of individual *sephirah* – attributes that represent aspects of life, of God and of ourselves. To study the Tree of Life through meditation is to explore and experience each *sephirah* in turn. In many ways, the layout of the *sephirah* in the Tree of Life corresponds to the positioning of the *chakra*s in the human body in Hindu tradition (see page 76).

CHAKRA MEDITATION

Spend time during your meditation sessions
acquainting yourself with your *chakra*s. Focus your
awareness on each *chakra* in turn and try to sense the
strength and goodness of its spinning energy. Begin at
the root *chakra* (situated at the base of your spine) and
work up through the sacral *chakra* (just beneath
your navel), solar plexus *chakra* (mid-stomach
area), heart *chakra*, throat *chakra*, third eye *chakra*
(located in your forehead, behind your eyes) and
ending with your crown *chakra*, which
lies just above your head.

TREE OF LIFE MEDITATION

Studying the Tree of Life during meditation can lead
us to greater self-awareness — the paths that link each
sephirah represent the different levels of our spiritual
development. Visualize these levels during your
meditation practice. Imagine that in doing so you are
reflecting on your own life's journey.

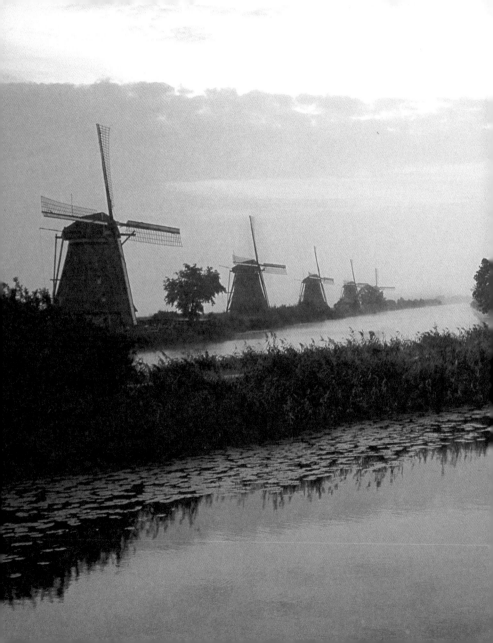

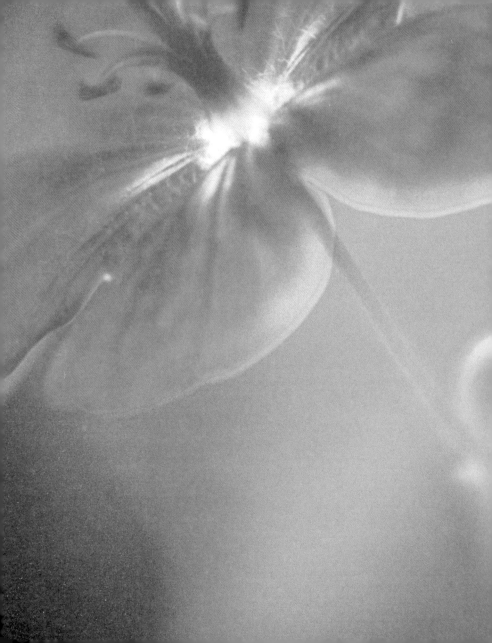

MEDITATE ON A FLOWER

This exercise uses a flower – a symbol of growth and achievement – to encourage the imagination to expand.

1 When you are comfortable and relaxed, picture a flower bud in your mind's eye. Contemplate what has led to the creation of this bud – the seed, the seedling, its nourishment by the sun and rain. Contemplate the potential in this flower bud, ready to open and reveal its beauty.

2 Imagine the bud slowly opening and becoming a full flower. Be creative in your vision, but don't force it – allow the bud to grow in your mind's eye as it wishes. Let the flower's colour, beauty and perfume fill you. Visualize fully the delicate nature of its petals.

3 Now think of the flower bud as representing something inside yourself that has been preparing to burst forth, such as loving compassion for others, or the strength to tackle a difficult situation. Meditate on the blossoming of the flower in your own life. Draw strength from your visualization and fulfil your own potential for growth.

EARTH'S ENERGY

The natural world provides a visual stimulus that
can have a powerful influence on the mind. Although
it may not always be possible to meditate on top of a
mountain or by the water's edge, such landscapes
are always easily accessible in our imagination. In
many religious traditions, mountains are viewed
as sacred places that form a link between heaven
and earth. The sea also holds great power and
symbolic significance – it is the origin of all life,
a metaphor for wisdom and a symbol of the
hidden depths of the unconscious. Calling upon
natural images such as these during meditation can
bring us closer in touch with our spiritual selves.

SOUND AND MEDITATION

The most fundamental way in which we apprehend and assess the world around us is by using our sense of sight. In the preceding pages we have talked a lot about visual symbols and the use of our imagination in meditation — and most people can engage immediately with this approach. But our sense of hearing is also crucially important in meditation, and it is well worth learning about the effect that different sounds can have in helping to focus attention and encourage a meditative state.

It is often assumed that successful meditation requires silent surroundings. This is indeed helpful if you are just beginning your meditation journey; but sometimes a certain level of background noise can be just as conducive to meditation practice as no sound at all. If you find the noise level becomes intrusive during meditation, tell yourself that the sounds you hear will take you deeper into your meditation, helping you to relax more completely. Try to turn what you may at first experience as a negative influence into a positive one.

NATURE'S SYMPHONY

Many people find that the symphonies of the natural world – the sounds of the sea, a breeze, trickling water, and rustling leaves, as well as the melodies of birdsong and the musical calling of dolphins or whales – have a calming influence over them and help them to attain a deep meditative state. This is probably because we have an in-built, fundamental connection with nature. Experiment to see which of nature's sounds work best for you. For example, the sound of waves crashing on a shoreline may be relaxing to one person, but to another may be stressful and even frightening. You can easily obtain audio tapes, CDs, or mini-disks of natural sounds and, when appropriate, it is well worth using these as a focus for your meditation sessions.

Give it a go! Next time you go for a country walk, fill your mind with the sounds of nature – give your undivided attention to each sound you hear. As you do so, remind yourself of the deep sense of connection with the natural world which lies at the core of your being.

REPETITIVE SOUND AND TRANCE

People sometimes question whether the use of
repetitive sound during meditation can induce a
hypnotic, trance-like state in the practitioner. Trance
can only be induced if either the use of repetitive sound
is extreme (in other words, if it is loud, overwhelming
and continues for long periods) or if the practitioner is
highly suggestible and easily influenced (if this is you
then it may not be a good time to meditate – wait until
you are feeling more at ease within yourself). In
normal circumstances, the practitioner should be in
full control of what he or she experiences during
meditation, and able to stop at any point if so desired.

FALLING ASLEEP

Most people discover that tiredness disappears
during meditation, but some find that listening to
soothing sounds – such as falling rain – puts them
to sleep while practising. If this happens to you,
reserve listening to soporific sounds until
last thing at night.

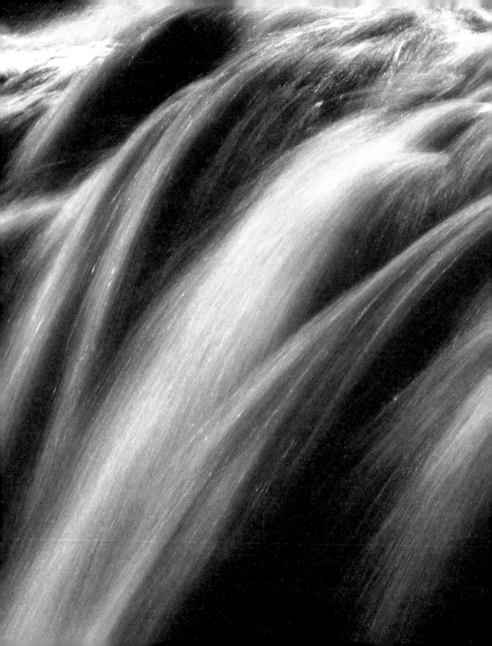

THE POWER OF MANTRAS

According to Eastern thought, all things are composed of vibrating energies. These vibrations are like sounds – in Hinduism creation itself is said to have been started by the primal sound *Om*. When a meditator takes up chanting, the chant is believed to influence the vibrations in his or her own body, and bring about a deep sense of well-being. A *mantra* is a word or phrase that is said to contain spiritual powers when chanted. There are several ancient *mantra*s that have been in use for centuries, such as the Buddhist chant *Om mani padme hum*. This *mantra* describes the jewel in the lotus of the heart, and it is a way of expressing the divinity that lies at the core of every human being.

It is thought by some that *mantra*s are effective because the mind is infinitely suggestible. Indeed, we often give ourselves the wrong "message" by telling ourselves that we "can't" or "won't" do something. For this reason, it is important that you choose your *mantra* carefully – when you chant in meditation, you are feeding your unconscious mind with the message contained within the *mantra*. Make sure that your *mantra* is a positive affirmation or, at the very least, a reminder of what it is that you wish to achieve. Any words that have significance for you can be used or adapted for chanting – the words used need not be esoteric or incomprehensible.

Traditionally, a meditation teacher will provide his or her student with a suitable *mantra* – a good teacher is able to recognize what is appropriate for their student at any given time. If you are your own teacher, seek out your *mantra* wisely. Perhaps a phrase in a spiritual text has resonance for you – you could use this; or you might have a deep calling to chant for peace, humility or kindness in your life. Even a simple word, such as "tranquillity" can be a *mantra*.

The exercise on page 93 shows you how to meditate using a *mantra*. At first, it may feel unnatural or uncomfortable to chant, but with time and practice, you may find that the *mantra* becomes an accepted and precious part of your meditation practice and that its positive effects become tangible in your life.

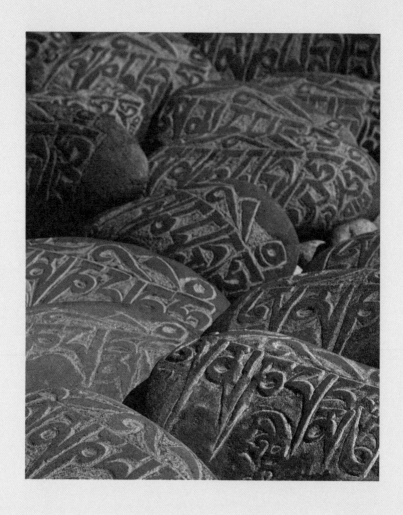

CHANTING A MANTRA

This exercise will help you to feel comfortable with your chosen *mantra*. Initially, aim to chant for five minutes or so – any longer and you may find that the effect becomes too trance-like and you begin to lose focus.

1   Sit comfortably and close your eyes. Focus your attention on your breathing – it should be relaxed, regular and a little deeper than normal.

2   Say your *mantra* to yourself a few times. When you are ready, say it out loud (try to keep your voice soft but clearly audible). Try to be aware of the sounds the words make – don't worry about their meaning. Keep your breathing deep and steady. Continue repeating your *mantra* for about five minutes.

3   When you feel ready, stop chanting and return your attention to your breathing once more. Can you feel the vibrations of the sound echoing through you? If so, spend a few moments simply enjoying this experience.

Speak to me of lovely things, of treasures yet
to be found, of peace that flows like a river.
Tell me of tranquil places that no hand has
marred, no storm has scarred. Give me
visions of standing in the sunlight, or feeling
the mist against my cheek as I move and live
and breathe ... . Find me a place in the sun
to sit and think and listen to the sweet inner
voice that says so quietly, "Peace. Be still."

JOYCE SEQUICHIE HIFLER
WHEN THE NIGHT BIRD SINGS (20TH CENTURY)

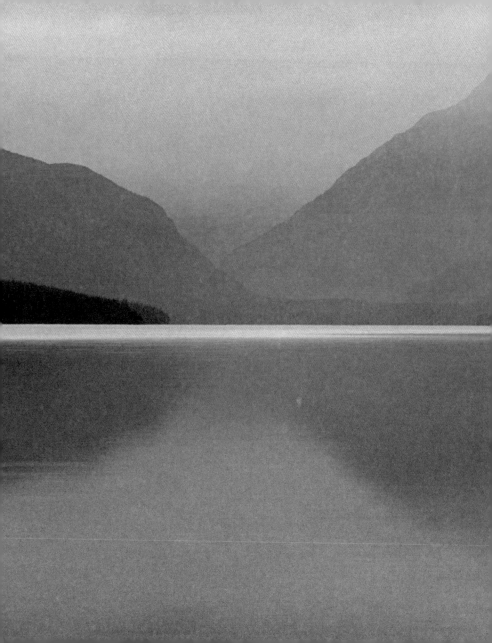

AFFIRMATIONS

Unconscious thoughts can have a negative effect on us, undermining our ability to achieve our goals. The use of affirmations in meditation is a means of combatting and counteracting such negative influences in our lives. Choose an affirmation that is appropriate for you and use it as if it were a *mantra*. For example, it could be a purely practical affirmation that helps you to overcome a fear, such as taking an exam or going to the dentist, or it could be a general suggestion to the unconscious (as shown in the examples below). Try to make your affirmation as specific as possible. For example, rather than saying simply "I am able to achieve my goal," define what your goal is.

"I am happy, healthy and full of energy."
"I welcome kindness, honesty and peace into my life."
"I can do better than I have ever done before."
"I am not afraid to face my fears."
"Life is joyful and my life is a success."

TUNING IN

Music is meaningful sound that possesses structure, harmony and rhythm. It can be a means of expressing the inexpressible, of penetrating the depths of human nature. Our brains respond readily to the language of music and, just like natural sounds (see page 87), it can provide a perfect background for focusing the mind, setting a mood and creating positive associations. The influence of certain forms of music on the unconscious mind has been well documented: for example, carefully selected extracts from Mozart have often been used to stimulate creativity or to reduce stress – this phenomenon is known as the "Mozart Effect".

Listening to your favourite composer during meditation can reveal facets of the music that may previously have gone unnoticed. Music that expresses religious sentiment – from Gregorian chant and the mathematical musical structures of Bach in Western culture, to the long, winding hymns of praise found in classical Indian sitar music – can be a powerful and spiritually enlightening experience. But whatever your choice, it is important to distinguish the difference between meditating on the music and purely relaxing to it.

Try selecting extracts from pieces of music that you like and making your own recordings. Experiment with dubbing natural sounds so that you can combine both natural and compositional effects. You could try using music in combination with an affirmation (see page 96) – doing so may help to improve your confidence and your belief that you will achieve your goals. You may also find that meditating to music improves your memory and powers of concentration. Playing music during your meditation sessions can also create a mystical atmosphere which can take you into a deeper meditative state.

In order to overcome their nerves, actors and performers often focus their minds completely on one single aspect of their performance and try not to worry about anything else. This is a good technique for achieving a "successful" meditation. Focus on one thing only – in this case, the sound of the music – and simply let the rest take care of itself. It works!

A MOMENT'S REFLECTION

Now that our meditation journey is well under way, it may be useful to revisit and reiterate some key ideas that will help us progress smoothly along our path. The first reminder is of the importance of becoming an observer of ourselves and of all that goes on in our minds and bodies, including our inward experiences of image and sound. Although we may seem to have separated the observer from the observed, it is crucial in meditation to realize that any apparent separation is simply part of a process – initially, we focus independently on our mental and physical experiences, and then we recombine them. Ultimately, the observer and the observed are one and the same thing – one cannot exist without the other. This is the true meaning of the word "mindfulness" (see pages 46–7). When the mind is completely still, we become mindful of this sense of unity and wholeness.

Meditators often spend endless hours in pursuit of a state of oneness. But another crucial point we should take note of here is that it would be wrong to tick off the benefits of meditation as if they were its goals, the expected pay-off. The trick is that it should be effortless and come naturally. In Zen, the student who is learning to achieve a goal, is taught that one way to do this is to deliberately aim away from the goal! The message here is: practise, but do not have any expectations of success. If meditation is undertaken in a spirit of relaxed open-mindedness, you will find that, paradoxically, you will eventually achieve your goal. You will discover that you meditate purely for its own sake and not for the sake of any particular end result. When this happens, you will reap the greatest physical, mental and spiritual benefits from your meditation.

Finally, another essential factor in learning to meditate is that of timing – and this is also a matter of awareness and of patience. Don't force anything, or meditate when it is inappropriate for you to do so, such as when you have a lot of commitments and are unable to find time for yourself. Allow circumstances to change until they are conducive to meditation – reduce the effort involved by going with the natural rhythm of your life.

Chapter Four

self and beyond

Meditation is a path to happiness, contentment and enlightenment. But to attain such states we have first to recognize the spiritual dimension deep within ourselves and to incorporate it into our daily lives – if we deny this aspect of our existence, life becomes meaningless. We learn how to draw upon our spiritual inventory through meditation, how to develop a sense of belonging rather than alienation, a sense of purpose rather than point-lessness, a sense of pattern rather than chaos, and a sense of freedom rather than of imprisonment in a world beyond our control.

Meditation brings an awareness of these possibili-ties into our lives, and it does so by way of paradox: in order to achieve one thing we are sometimes taught to do the exact opposite – for example, to relax a muscle, we are encouraged to tense it first. Meditation teachings are full of such paradoxes – perhaps best exemplified by the Zen *koan* (see pages 104–105) – which aim to disrupt our tendency to encounter the world as polarized or dualistic. We learn, instead, to think not simply in terms of "either/or" but in terms of "both": we possess spiritual and material dimensions, inner and outer worlds, minds and bodies. In showing us how to dissolve the boundaries between such oppositions, meditation provides a means to spiritual growth that can make our lives unified, meaningful and sacred.

THE PARADOX OF THE KOAN

The *koan* is one of the principle teaching methods in the Rinzai school of Zen Buddhism and it is used to train the mind to attain enlightenment. A *koan* consists of a riddle, which at first glance has no apparent answer, or of a nonsensical or paradoxical question or statement. The most famous *koan* is, "What is the sound of one hand clapping?" Zen teachers assign *koans* to their students to help them break away from their normal patterns of thinking about and apprehending the world.

The significance of the *koan* lies not in finding a solution to the conundrum, but in engaging with our response to the intellectual impasse that arises in our minds when we contemplate it. This new way of seeing, this simple yet ultimate realization toward which the *koan* points, can guide us in our daily lives. One of the intentions of meditation is the healing of opposites — and this is precisely what the Zen *koan* also strives to achieve. Its conundrums indicate an underlying unity of opposites, and although the initial intention may be to break up traditional patterns of thought, its principle aim is to point toward wholeness.

The *koan*, as with other meditation practices, leads ultimately to enlightenment, or perhaps something just short of it. During this process, it may appear that an outer layer of reality has been peeled away in order to reveal something profound and miraculous beneath. But, according to Zen, herein lies a danger. The Zen teacher will gently steer the pupil away from this experience of the miraculous (which is referred to by the word *makyo*) firmly back to the practice of meditation and will suggest that the miracle of life is "doing the dishes and putting out the garbage" – the miracle lies not so much in being able to walk on water but, quite simply, in being able to walk.

In meditation, we should be careful to ensure that our feet are always planted firmly on the ground: no matter how great our insights and experiences may be, life goes on unchanged. The Zen *koan* is a powerful device but, ultimately, it consists merely of a few words – nothing more and nothing less.

WHO AM I?

Amid the pressures of the modern world, "finding our-selves", attempting to discover our true identity, has become an important goal. Meditation can often encourage us to focus on the great questions of life, such as, "Who am I?" This single question gives rise to many others: "What is my purpose?", "How do I fit in with the great scheme of things?", "Do I possess freedom in life?", "Where have I come from?", "Where am I going?" These questions are like *koan*s (see pages 104–105) – they have no simple, clear-cut answers, but the mere asking of them opens up possibilities that had not existed previously, taking us away from ignorance toward insight, understanding and enlightenment. In practising meditation you will not suddenly and mira-culously be transformed into a completely different individual – rather, the person you *already* are, your real identity, will gradually become apparent to you.

Western culture emphasizes our individuality, our separateness from one another – it is an emphasis which can have a profoundly isolating and alienating effect on us. As human beings, we have a physical, emotional, intellectual and spiritual existence. We are past, present and future. Our individual psyches have been formed from our memories and former experiences, from the things we have learned as well as the things we have forgotten. Above and beyond this, however, we contain within ourselves more than just our individuality: we belong to a race, to a history, to a civilization and, ultimately, to a process of evolution.

We are, then, individuals and yet we have a collective identity that we share with the rest of humanity. It is this common factor that meditation seeks to bring to our attention, for contained within it is the source of life energy (referred to in some traditions as *qi* or *prana*). In reaching out toward this energy, be aware that you are taking part in a great tradition. Meditation encourages us to recognize that we are part of a greater whole and offers us spiritual guidance on how to draw support and gain great inner strength and self-knowledge from this deep sense of belonging.

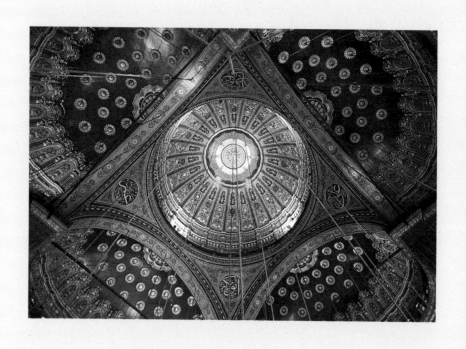

LETTING GO OF THE PAST

Letting go of the past allows us to learn, to grow and to change. This exercise will help you move forward in life.

1 Sit comfortably. Imagine that you are alone in an ancient, sacred temple. Call up your earliest memories – as far back into the recesses of your mind as you can go. Meditate upon these earliest memories and let them go, saying, "I release my past; I am ready to move on."

2 Now allow the memories of significant turning points in your life gradually to come to mind. Meditate on them one by one and then let them go, saying to yourself, "I release my past; I am ready to move on."

3 Tell yourself that the sacred space in which you imagine yourself represents your past. It is special to you, and is a place that you can visit whenever you choose to do so. Say to yourself, "I release my past; I am ready to move on." When you feel it is time to end the meditation, let the image of the temple fade from your mind.

The Self is omniscient, all-understanding,
and its glory manifests in the universe.
It is pure consciousness, dwelling in the
heart of all, in the divine city of Brahma.
There is no space it does not fill.
It is established deep within the mind,
and is the silent, vital force which guides the
body and the senses.
The wise obtain bliss and immortality
by beholding this Self, shining forth
through everything.

MUNDAKA UPANISHAD (c.800BCE–c.300BCE)

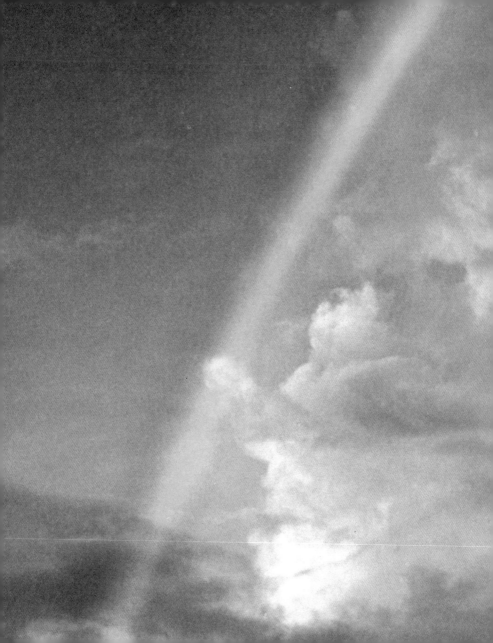

DISCOVERING YOUR TRUE NATURE

The Sanskrit word *buddha* originally meant "awakening" or "coming to". The word later took on the meaning of "spiritual awakening". Buddhists speak of our "*buddha*-nature", which is our true nature. The spiritual insights of the Buddha are most clearly expressed in his doctrine of the "Four Noble Truths". In this doctrine, which forms the basis of Buddhism, the Buddha diagnoses the human condition and also prescribes a treatment – the path toward *nirvana*. The Buddha's life-story reveals that it was through his realization of the Four Truths that he finally attained enlightenment. Only through an awareness of such universal truths in life, can we also arrive at an understanding of ourselves as individuals, of our own true nature.

The First Truth is that all mortal life involves suffering in the form of sickness, aging and death; the Second Truth insists that suffering is caused by desire; the Third Truth is that in eliminating desire, we eliminate our suffering; and the Fourth Truth offers a means of release from suffering: the "Eightfold Path", which identifies the eight factors that will lead to the end of suffering. These factors express the main elements of Buddhist training – moral conduct, concentration and wisdom.

Suffering can arise from our craving to be individual, and this affects everything that we see and do: our beliefs, our aims and aspirations, our morals and our attitudes to life and death. According to Buddhist philosophy, we are asleep in a dream world because we refuse to accept the reality of the universal truths that stare us in the face. We are not individuals, separate and self-contained, but part of a greater whole from which we were born and to which we will return when we die. Life is a brief moment in the totality of our true existence.

Meditation allows us to experience the infinite depth in ourselves and our interconnectedness with the world at large. Through meditation, we can come to an awareness of our true nature, and arrive at the realization that life is as it is. With this awakening, nothing changes, everything remains the same – apart from our attitudes and the way in which we conduct our lives.

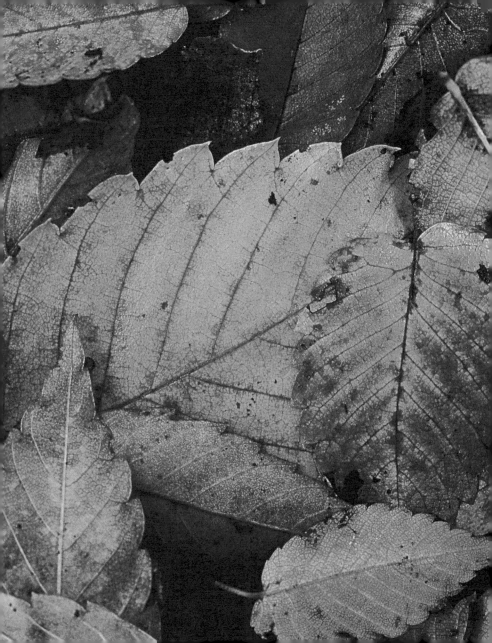

ACCEPTING CHANGE

Change means leaving the old behind and accepting the new into our lives: focus on this idea in the following meditation to help you to accept changes in your life.

1   Sit comfortably and close your eyes. Meditate on your feelings about change in a state of open-mindedness. Be ready to accept whatever comes to you.

2   Allow feelings and thoughts to come to you in response to your openness to change. Even if they are not thoughts and feelings that you like, try to develop a non-judgmental attitude toward them – focus your awareness on them for a moment, but do nothing else. Accept them and allow them to pass unhindered through your mind.

3   When you are ready, let these feelings go, leaving yourself in a state of readiness and heightened awareness, able to respond positively to what the future brings.

GO WITH THE FLOW

Changes are taking place in life all the time, and Taoist philosophy insists that we can gain strength and insight by accepting that the universe is in a constant state of flux and that there is a natural flow to life. According to the principles of Taoism, through meditation we are able to discover the direction of this natural flow and move with it. We should not waste our time and energy attempting to struggle against it. Sometimes the flow suggests doing nothing, sometimes acting, sometimes changing, sometimes remaining the same. This is the essence of the Tao.

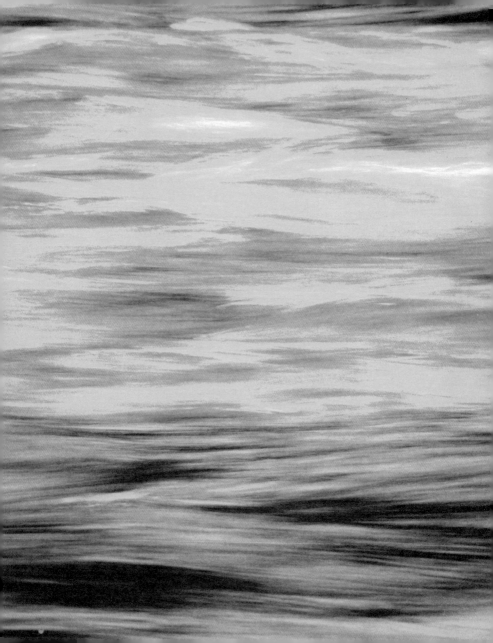

THE INTERCONNECTEDNESS
OF ALL THINGS

In the West, we are often taught as children to observe the universe "objectively" – this polarity of observer and observed is a necessary condition for a culture based on materialistic, scientific principles. But on an individual level, such a view of the world can leave us with a sense of separation, even isolation.

By contrast, many Eastern spiritual traditions suggest that we are connected with the external world in profound and fundamental ways – the themes of oneness, wholeness and interconnectedness are common in meditation. Mind and body, conscious and unconscious, internal and external are involved in a symbiotic relationship that affects the way in which we apprehend the world. It is not uncommon for people who meditate regularly to experience remarkable coincidences; such events, meetings or encounters become charged with meaning, as if they have been brought at the right time and place – nothing happens purely by chance.

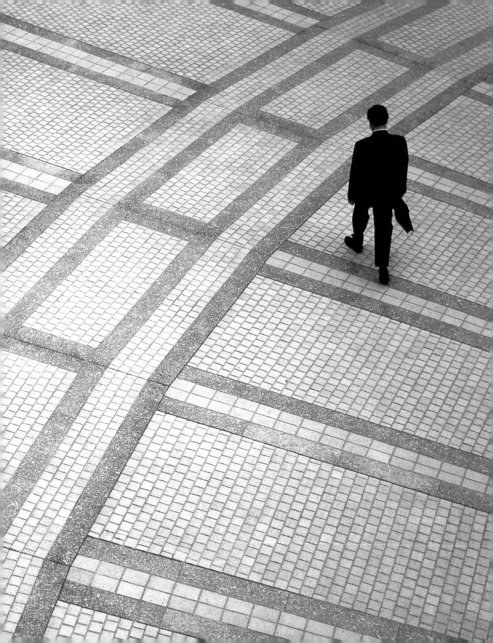

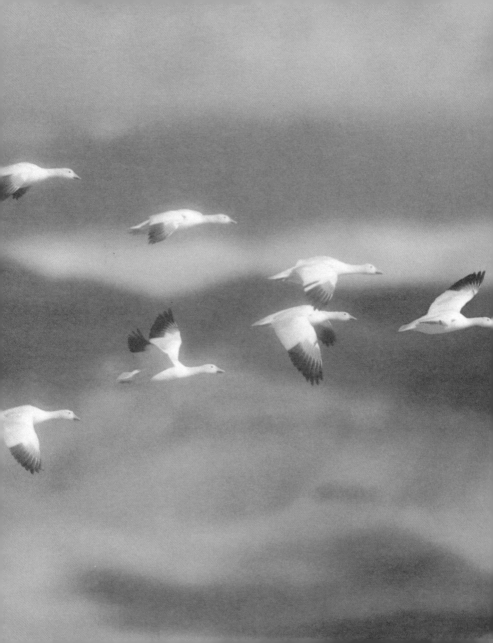

LOVING KINDNESS MEDITATION

The ability to love and to forgive are gifts of the spirit, available to us all. This meditation encourages you to practise outwardly what you experience inwardly.

1　Sit comfortably in your meditation position. Think back to any recent unkindnesses that have been done to you. Try not to dwell on the feelings you may have had as a result, simply recall the incident and let go.

2　Recall any unkind acts of your own toward others – don't dwell on how you felt, simply remember and let go.

3　Now meditate on the interconnectedness of all things. Say to yourself (out loud or in your head), "I forgive myself and others." Make a promise to yourself that in all your encounters you will try to transform any feelings of hurt or anger into understanding and loving kindness toward yourself and anyone else involved.

COMING FULL CIRCLE

We will finish our meditation journey where we began, by recalling what meditation is, and what it is not. Meditation is being, not doing. You may create the right conditions in which to practise – a quiet space, good posture – but meditation does not begin when you close your eyes, nor does it end when you open them again. It is an attitude of mind which involves self-reflection, and which you carry through with you into everyday life. Its techniques have been developed over thousands of years: if you are asked to do something by a meditation teacher (or even by this book) that at first you don't understand, just go along with it – its meaning will eventually become clear to you.

Above all, be sensitive to your inner needs, develop a sense of responsibility toward yourself and others, be humble before the riches of the inner worlds and respectful of the traditions that have offered us the means to attain enlightenment. Follow these guidelines, and in time your true nature will be revealed to you.

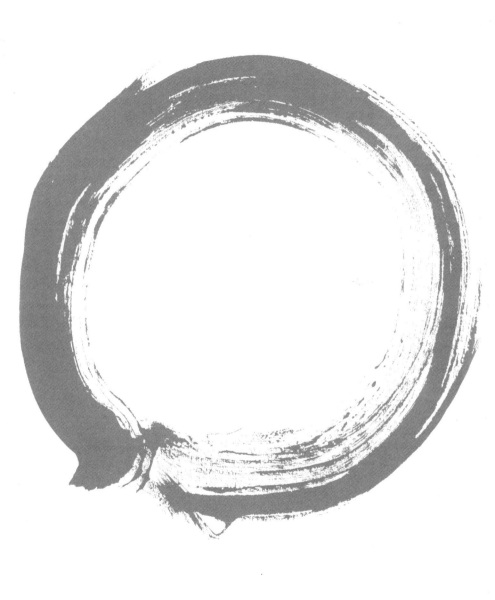

I want to beseech you ...
to be patient toward all
that is unsolved in your heart
and try to love the questions themselves
like locked rooms and
like books that are written in
a very foreign tongue.

Do not now seek the answers,
which cannot be given you
because you would not be
able to live them.
And the point is, to live everything.

Live the questions now.
Perhaps you will then
gradually, without noticing it,
evolve some distant day
into the answer.

RAINER MARIA RILKE

LETTERS TO A YOUNG POET (20TH CENTURY)

INDEX

The publisher would like to thank the following people, publishers, organizations, museums and photographic libraries for permission to reproduce their material (photographs and quotations). Every care has been taken to trace copyright holders. However, if we have omitted anyone we apologise and will, if informed, make corrections in any future editions of this book.

Picture Credits

Page 1 Photonica/Masao Ota; 2 Corbis/Philadelphia Museum of Art; 3 Corbis/Kevin R. Morris; 13 Corbis/Paul A. Souders; 18 Stone/Getty Images; 21 Photonica/William Huber; 23 Stone/Getty Images; 24 National Geographic Society Image Collection; 28 Photonica/Yukari Ochai; 31 Photonica/Ann Giordano; 34 National Geographic Society Image Collection; 37 DBP Archives; 38 Stone/Getty Images; 41 Bruce Coleman Collection; 48 Photonica/Knauer/Johnston; 51 Stone/Getty Images; 55 Stone/Getty Images; 58 Bruce Coleman Collection; 61 Corbis/CRD Photo; 63 Photonica/Neo Vision; 64 National Geographic Society Image Collection; 67 FPG/Getty Images; 71 Photonica/Ann Cutting; 72 The Art Archive; 74 Stone/Getty Images; 77 Charles Walker Collection; 78 The Art Archive; 81 The Photographer's Library; 82 Photonica/Miyoko Komine; 84 Stone/Getty Images; 89 Stone/Getty Images; 92 Corbis/Charles & Josette Lenars; 95 Bruce Coleman Collection; 97 Photonica/Chikara Amono; 108 Panos Pictures/Roderick Johnson; 111 Stone/Getty Images; 114 Photonica/Masao Ota; 117 Stone/Getty Images; 119 Photonica/Yoshini Tanaka; 120 Stone/Getty Images; 123 Yukki Yaura; 125 Photonica/Qwert Yui

Quotation Credits

p.36 Extract from "Buddha's Nature" by Wes Niker published by Rider, London. Used by permission of The Random House Group Limited.
p.60 Extract from "The Heart of the Buddha's Teachings" by Thich Nhat Hanh published by Rider, London. Used by permission of the Random House Group Limited.
p.66 "The Art of Peace" by Morihei Ueshiba, translated by John Stevens. © 1992 by John Stevens. Reprinted by arrangement with Shambhala Publications, Inc., Boston, www.shambhala.com
p.94 Extract from "When the Night Bird Sings" by Joyce Hifler, © Council Oak Books, Tulsa, 2000
p.124 Excerpted from "Letters to a Young Poet" by Rainer Maria Rilke, © 2000. Reprinted with permission of New World Library, Novato, CA 94949, www.newworldlibrary.com

Author's Acknowledgment

If thanks are due, they should be to the DBP team, for creating with me a book to be proud of!

Bill Anderton runs the Pilgrims Mind Body Spirit Centre in Gloucester. He is also author of the meditation tape "Crystal Clear". Information about the centre and tape can be found by visiting the website http://pilgrims.inetc.net or by sending an SAE to Pilgrims, College Court, Gloucester, GL1 2NJ.